Nursing School
Tips in A Nutshell

Nursing School Tips in A Nutshell

Olivia Nwaokeleme-Ekperikpe

To order additional copies of this book, contact:
Xlibris
844-714-8691
www.Xlibris.com
Orders@Xlibris.com
828549

Contents

Acknowledgement

This work will not be complete without acknowledging the special people that helped to make this possible. I will begin by thanking God for his grace, love, kindness, provisions and wisdom, Lian Liu who swapped her day shift with me for my night, for a full year to enable me to go to school in the morning, even though she did not like working nights, she did it for me. Mark Schriever, who taught me the basic things I needed to know about nursing as a novice, he made himself available for my questions, which sometimes were dumb, but he was stable and always there to provide answers. Anh Pham my moral support and my entire AIG assistance and medical crew, you guys were awesome. Boniface Nnaji for being my financial support when I could not meet up any longer, Eng. & Dr. Mrs. Nwabuoku for being there for me, supporting me financially and morally, Pastor Degorl and the entire Throne Room Church for praying for me, Mrs. Pearl Oguchi for making sure I ate well during a difficult time when I could not cook, my instructors for impacting knowledge. I thank everyone that impacted my life directly and indirectly during my nursing program. I will not forget to thank those that did not believe in me, those that thought I will not make it, thanks for being one of the forces that drove me to the finish line.

Dedication

This book is dedicated to the smart ladies and gentlemen who have devoted their lives to giving back to society by caring holistically for people who suffer from different kinds of sicknesses. They have devoted their lives and passion to loving the patients as their own and being the patients advocate. Thank you for all that you do as nurses.

Forward

This book provides tips on what to expect in the nursing program. It is an 'easy-to-pick-up-and-read' handbook that provides students with guidelines on how to manage their time and studies while in the program. Information is knowledge and as the saying goes, "Knowledge is power." I have derived enormous joy and pride in writing this book and I have extensive knowledge of nursing school. This is because I have personally gone through the nursing program and I am writing from experience. My utmost hope is that this book will be beneficial to nursing students as they follow these Nursing School Commandments and guidelines.

Introduction

This book was inspired by the struggles my classmates and I faced in nursing school. I realized that before going into the nursing program I had no idea how rigorous it would be. I had been in school all my life but by no means had I been in a program as hectic as the nursing program. My classmates and I faced many challenges and were compelled to seek solutions by purchasing books that would help direct us through the program. That was when this idea was born. Being an author, I took it upon myself as my joy and privilege to share my nursing school experience with others who plan to enter the program and may have an inkling of what to expect but lack in-depth knowledge of the intricacies and rigors of the program.

Nursing school is exhausting. It can drain your energy, but with good management of time and resources you can achieve success. The nursing school experience can become a win-win situation for all – the students, their proud families and the school. This book covers what I call the Twelve Commandments of Nursing School which students must follow to help them get through the difficult process of accomplishing this great academic achievement.

Chapter One

EXPECTATIONS OF NURSING SCHOOL

Hurray! You made it into nursing school, now what? You think the long hours of studying, getting your prerequisites done and passing your entrance exam have paid off and now you can relax. No way! You have just started. Going through nursing school is like a baby learning how to sit, crawl and walk. The stage of completing your prerequisites can be compared to the stage at which a baby learns to sit up on her own. When you get into the nursing program, you will have to learn which particular movement technique works best for you since everyone is different. You may have to learn how to crawl on the floor using your abdomen or your knees, whichever method works best for you; it does not matter the technique used. What is important is that you learn how to sit and crawl in your first semester of nursing school (which can be likened to your baby crawling stage).

Your baby crawling stage is your stepping stone to learning how to walk. In time, as you get comfortable with your crawling skills you begin to learn how to walk. At first, it makes no sense as you wobble and fall. These are the times when you have studied for your test but only make a low grade and yet do not give up. This is just like a child who falls so many times in learning how to walk but still gets up and tries to walk again. With time the child will learn how to walk erectly without falling, and so will you if you persevere. If you persevere, you will be able to turn those grades around, stand firm in the program and even learn to run. Remember that if you fail any class in nursing school you will have to repeat that class. If you fail it a second time, you will be kicked out of the program, no mercies; that is the rule in most schools (please check your school policy).

Once you enter the nursing program there are rigid rules and regulations that you must follow to enable you achieve the success that you desire. I have laid out the Twelve Commandments of Nursing School below.

Twelve Commandments of Nursing School

1. Nursing school is the avenue that will transform your life for the better
2. You shall place your studies first and not be distracted by other activities
3. You shall not let family or friends disrupt your studies
4. You shall make sure you have a good support system
5. You shall take your studies seriously and not lightly
6. Remember that your input will determine your output
7. Honor schedules by being punctual to class and clinical
8. You shall not miss clinical unless for very serious, genuine reasons
9. You shall not submit your assignments even a second late

10. You shall tackle and review many sample questions

11. Remember to ask questions when you don't understand

12. You shall find positive ways to take good care of yourself and maintain good health during the course of the program.

The decision to apply to nursing school was not born overnight. That I know because you have to complete your prerequisite courses and make sure you have a high GPA to qualify you to enter into nursing school. Nursing school is highly competitive and schools only choose the best students to represent them because, success in the nursing board exam reflects on the school. For you to have decided to go to nursing school, you must have thought it through and known for certain in your heart that nursing is the profession you want to pursue. Different people have different reasons for desiring to go into nursing. Some people go into nursing because they would like to care for people and give back to society, while some actually go into the profession just for the financial benefit. However, I have to tell you this: you really need to ask yourself,

"Why am I going to nursing school?" If you are going into nursing just for financial reasons, you will end up being a horrible nurse and will not be in the profession very long. You must have the passion, empathy, compassion, patience and a good communication skill and more, to become a nurse. Some of these qualities mentioned will enable you to become successful as a nurse. Your compassion, empathy, the desire to give back to the society, the tendency to not be judgmental or inconsiderate, and being a good listener, will take you a long way in nursing. You must be ready to always put your clients above any personal prejudices you may hold. Nursing is not an easy profession. You really need to examine your motives before going into it.

Chapter Two

NURSING SCHOOL IS THE AVENUE THAT WILL TRANSFORM YOUR LIFE FOR THE BETTER

Different people may have different desires for entering the nursing program, but the end goal for all is that the decision to pursue nursing will pave a path or an avenue for a better life. Some people who go into the nursing program have been in different job fields that did not give them fulfillment. They believe that converting to the nursing profession will provide them with a fulfilling job that will always be in demand and that will secure their future.

The earlier you realize that being in the nursing

program is the gateway to the future you have always desired, the better it will be for you. This will enable you focus on achieving your goals. The pathway to achieving your goals is not smooth. You will surely have a bumpy ride and go through some very scary routes, but if you persevere through all these you will overcome.

You have to set your goals and in your imagination place your future title as "RN" as the ultimate reward that will keep driving you to achieve your set goals. You should do everything in your power to achieve your goals because, though the resources to attain them will be provided for you, you are the sole author of your future in the nursing program. As the saying goes, "When the going gets tough, the tough get going."

The pathway to achieving your goals is going to be rough. There will be times when you will feel like giving up, but in those times remember your utmost goal – the RN badge that you will wear on your scrubs when you are working as a registered nurse. Some people are visual, and if you are the visual type you can buy any object that you like and consider it to be a good inspiration piece to place in your study area. It will be a symbol of the prize you will win when you graduate from nursing school.

Once you graduate you will be able to get a well-paid job that will allow you to live a better and more fulfilled life doing the job you love. There is great joy in working in a field or profession that you love.

Chapter Three

YOU SHALL PLACE YOUR STUDIES FIRST AND NOT BE DISTRACTED BY OTHER ACTIVITIES

This is the time to put your game gear on, no room for play and no room for procrastination. The assignments will be overwhelming, not to mention the numerous pages of reading that you will have to cover for your next exam. You have a decision to make at this point, which is to make your studies your priority and pass your exams, or allow yourself to be distracted by social media and other activities going on around you. There is a price to pay to achieve your goal.

To achieve your goal, you must be a little selfish in the

sense that you must choose to forego other commitments and devote almost all your time to studying and doing your school work. For those of you who have a husband and children, let them know that you love them but must still make your studies your priority for this period of time. Explain to them what the winning prize will be at the end of the tunnel – a better future for the entire family! You will still have to make out time somehow to be with your children and husband occasionally, though it will not be as frequent as before. Otherwise, your children might think you are abandoning them, especially if they are young and cannot understand the sacrifices you are making. Continuously let them know that you love them and that you are in school, which is why you always have to study and cannot spend quality time with them.

Placing your studies first will allow you to focus on what is necessary and give you the mental clarity you need to map out the right studying strategy, that is, the unique style that suits you and you alone. You may be the type who reads the whole chapter and bookmarks or highlights the sentences that strike you as important. On the other hand, you may be the type who reads and stores information by making flash cards. You may even be the type who reads and makes notes. Whichever technique works best for you, go ahead and implement it so far as it gets you a passing grade. If you adopt a certain technique that you find does not work for you, ask other students for suggestions on how they study and try out another technique. It might actually work for you. I personally read the whole chapter and highlight the important sentences and then go back to review those highlights two to three times before the exam.

Regarding tests and examinations, there are different types of testing or different question types. There is the 'multiple select' question type – the 'select-all-that-apply' question type. This requires you to really know the core content of the topic that you are being tested on. Consequently, you would need to review each chapter very well. A good technique to use in 'select-all-that-apply' testing is to consider if each option is true or false. If the option does not apply to the question, it might not be the correct answer. Then there are multiple choice questions in which four different options are provided as answers for each question from which you are required to choose the correct answer. At times, all four options may be correct but one may be the most correct or the most accurate. You are therefore, required to know the core content thoroughly so that you do not harbor any doubts regarding which option is the most accurate. This would enable you to select the right answer, the specific answer that is required.

A helpful study tool is to engage in group study. You may align yourself with a group that you can work positively with. You must try as much as possible to avoid the negative. You may encounter negativity if you pair up with the wrong person or the wrong group. It would be very toxic to work within such an environment. Once you find the ideal study group, make it a point for the group to assign a reading or allocate an assignment to each person. That way when you converge everyone will be able to participate and contribute effectively to the group. I can tell you from experience that it is very rewarding to be in a study group because there are particular things another person will state that will ring a bell in your memory during the exam and help you pick the correct answer.

In nursing school, you will surely burn the midnight candle as they say. Most times, you will find yourself studying into the wee hours of the morning while everyone else is asleep. Coffee and tea will be your partners in your efforts to stay awake. Do persevere because you will overcome and certainly be glad when you have jumped the hurdle of passing your exams. You will forget all the sleepless nights you spent studying and only remember the joy of passing. In the event you fail an exam, you will need to encourage yourself by telling yourself and believing that you will do better on the next exam. There are usually about three to four exams in a semester depending on which school you attend. If you fail an exam, make sure you schedule a review of the exam with your instructor. That way you can find out where your weaknesses are and ask your instructor how you could do better.

I do believe that with more effort you can make it; several of us have made it through different difficult circumstances. I remember when a couple of my classmates did not do great on a particular exam in our final semester and almost gave up. I encouraged them not to give up and asked what score they needed to make on the next exam in order to get an overall passing grade. They needed to make a score of 86%. I encouraged them to study and assured them it was possible to make that grade on the next exam. They laughed at me and thought I was crazy. One of them even told me, "You say it so casually as if making an 86 on the exam is easy. I made a 56 on the last exam. Do you really think I will be able to make 86 on the next one?"

My answer without a doubt was "Yes!" I assured them that having *determination* and *zeal* was the key. On the next exam they surely did make 86% and even more than that because they were determined to succeed. After receiving their scores, they happily confirmed to me that they had made it.

It was a thing of joy to see that they made it. So, one thing I have to bring to attention is fact that being in nursing school, you are not in competition with anyone. When you applied to nursing school you probably did not know any of your classmates. Therefore, see yourselves as comrades and be there for each other. It does not matter if you have an A or a C in nursing school, both those who had an A and a C will ultimately graduate and guess what? You might not see each other again in life after graduation. So why compete? I will advise you to bring a positive attitude towards your colleagues. Rejoice and sympathize with each other, do not hoard information. United, you and your classmates will excel. Ask yourself this question; "How would people remember me after nursing school?" However way you want people to remember you, then carry yourself that way throughout the program and help other students when you can.

Chapter Four

YOU SHALL NOT LET FAMILY OR FRIENDS DISRUPT YOUR STUDIES

We all know the saying "no man is an island". However, during nursing school you must plan to become an island by isolating yourself from family distractions. I advise that you sit down with all parties involved to explain your reasons for isolating yourself. Let them know you love them very much but are doing this because you want a better and brighter future for yourself and your family. It is important for you to know that many families suffer when a parent, girlfriend or boyfriend enroll in nursing school. From what

I observed, many break ups in relationships and marriages occurred during the course of the nursing program. It really did not have to be so. There were still many relationships that survived the challenges of nursing school. One person I know had to drop out of the nursing program because her marriage was about to break up and she valued her marriage more than the nursing school. You need to assess your family well and know how best to handle them. You must let them understand the reason why you are doing what you are doing.

There will be activities and games that you will miss out on within this period of time; there will be parties you will be unable to attend. However, when you are done with school you can party all you want and go to any game that you would like to attend. Your main focus at this time should be your academic goal, how to achieve it and the right measures to take to ensure that you achieve your goal. When you isolate yourself to study, make sure you are really studying and not just pretending to study as you will only end up deceiving yourself. You must understand that a lot is at stake.

Family is very important. Even though you must isolate

yourself so that you can study, I advise that you make out a special day and time to devote to your husband alone and a special time for your children as well. Make sure you let them understand that they are loved and that you do not intend to push them away. This is very important and will even enable everyone else in the family to take up your responsibilities and free up your time to allow you to study. I know that with many of my female nursing school colleagues who were married their husbands took over their chores to give them ample time to study. Today, they have graduated from nursing school and have passed their board exam. A brighter future awaits them. Yeah! If you are single, the nursing school period may seem very long for you as well because the time you formerly allotted to dating will suffer. You must understand however, that once you graduate you will have all the time to resume dating. If you are already in a committed relationship, your partner will still love you even if you are not as available as you were before, if the love is real. Your main focus at this stage should be your studies. Do not let friends and family disrupt your study time.

Chapter Five

YOU SHALL MAKE SURE YOU HAVE A GOOD SUPPORT SYSTEM

Having a good support system is a tremendous help and will alleviate some of the burdens you will encounter as a student, especially if you are a mother, spouse or even a grandparent who is responsible for raising your child, children or grandchildren. Yes, some nursing school students are grandparents, and they should be applauded for their courage to pursue this particular goal they have set for themselves. I personally think it is amazing and worthy of emulation.

During nursing school, there will be many times when you will be buried in your books. Your children may not be able to see you as often as they used to as you may find yourself stuck in the library after school due to a deadline you have to meet. It would be a relief to have a support system that you can rely on like your husband, parents or parents-in-law, aunts, uncles and friends who would be willing to pick your child or children up from school or take them to games if you are in clinical or class. You will need someone to make sure they have had something to eat and someone who will help them with their homework and tuck them into bed.

Students who are fortunate to have a good support system end up having a more relaxed mind and are able to study better. However, before you begin the program and become increasingly absent from home, you need to explain to your children why mommy or daddy will not be home as often as before. Let them know how much you love them and explain that you will be in school and often absent from them so they do not feel abandoned and unloved. You never know what goes on in the minds of these little ones and I cannot overemphasize this point; it is very important.

Remember to be appreciative of your support system. Let them know how glad you are that they are there for you, not just with words but also in action by making sure you excel in your academics, that way, the time they sacrifice supporting you will not be in vain. Remember that you will still have to make a little bit of time for family, no matter how little that time is. Do not zone out completely. Why am I saying this? I am saying this because many families go through crisis during the nursing school period. Some relationships break up while others stand the test of time. You must work hard to ensure that you are communicating effectively with your partner and children by continuously letting them know that you love them and that this hectic time will not last for eternity; it will only be for a period of time. Appreciate every support you get; it will help soothe some of the anxiety you will face as a student.

Chapter Six

YOU SHALL TAKE YOUR STUDIES
SERIOUSLY AND NOT LIGHTLY

Nursing school is serious business. You may have come in with a **GPA** of 3.9 or even 4.0. However, if you do not take care you may leave with a **GPA** of 2.9. That is how difficult nursing school is. I am saying this to let you know that you cannot afford to take your studies lightly. You may be used to getting all A's on your exams but in nursing school you may find yourself getting a B, C or even failing the exam altogether.

The questions on tests and exams are not ordinary

questions; they are not direct questions. There is a technique to answering them. You need to learn the right technique for answering questions by using your critical thinking abilities. It is very easy for you to provide the wrong answer on a question whose subject matter you are familiar with because of the way the question is phrased. It is imperative that you buy the necessary study materials that will help you develop the correct technique. I remember panicking after my second semester Medical-Surgical (Med-Surg) Exam. Even though I passed it, I was not used to getting a C. I was so desperate that I actually reached out directly to Elsevier to ask which resource would help me develop my critical thinking abilities. Elsevier is a publishing company that specializes in scientific and medical resource material. I was advised to purchase "Saunders Strategies for Test Success: Passing Nursing School and the NCLEX Exam." This resource really helped me better understand how to answer questions.

No matter how many books on testing you read to help you better understand how to answer questions, ultimately the ball is in your court to pass your exams. It rests on you to take your studies seriously; it rests on you to study with understanding and to retain what you have studied and to correctly apply it when you are in the exam. Your ultimate goal is to pass each exam. In my time, the passing grade when we started nursing school was seventy percent. Many of us were struggling to make that grade when to our surprise the school hiked up the passing grade to seventy-five percent. At first it made no sense as people were already struggling to pass. The actual reason the school raised the passing grade was to set a higher academic standard for students and force them to raise their grades so that they would not struggle to pass the nursing board exam. Nursing schools want you to be solid and well-equipped for the board exam. If you are well-prepared you will represent them well when you take the **NCLEX-RN** (National Council Licensure Examination-Registered Nurse). Yes, you are being drilled to pass nursing school, but ultimately the school's goal is to make sure that you are ready for your board exam. During the nursing program, your main focus should be to ensure that you are taking your studies seriously and not wasting your time with irrelevant things. Learn the core content of what you are being taught and you will do well. My advice is that you study hard to pass your exams the first time, endeavor to concentrate on your school exams before you think of **NCLEX**. You may ask why am saying this. I say this because I knew someone who in our first year of nursing school, was busy studying **NCLEX** questions and was very good at it but neglected to study for the current nursing courses and that individual failed out of nursing school. Therefore, concentrate first and pass your nursing school exams that will propel you to graduate, once you graduate from nursing school, I believe you are already equipped to pass your **NCLEX**.

Chapter Seven

REMEMBER THAT YOUR INPUT WILL DETERMINE YOUR OUTPUT

You should be aware that your input will determine your output in the nursing program and generally with most things in life. As I said earlier, you need to take your studies seriously to enable you achieve the ultimate goal, which is to graduate from nursing school. Nursing school is the gateway to a better future. To attain that goal you will have to work hard. Nursing is not a program you can come into and think you can succeed by merely memorizing information.

I remember when in the first semester of the program one of our instructors told us that the content we were learning would not make sense to us at that point, but that the knowledge we were acquiring would build up and we would understand it all by the time we graduated. It was very true. Most students who enter the nursing program do so fresh from high school or switch to nursing from other careers and some do have medical background. I am one such example. I have a Bachelor's degree in Business Management, worked in the cooperate world and I had no medical background whatsoever. In the first semester, I had no idea what 'dysphagia' was. When I look back on things, I simply laugh because I definitely know what 'dysphagia' is now. When I got a question about stomatitis in the exam of my first semester, I thought stomatitis had something to do with the stomach. How ignorant! This is simply to let you know that though you may come into the nursing program as a novice, you will acclimatize to the program but you will have to work hard by putting productive hours into studying. You cannot just rely on doing your class work; you have to tackle NCLEX questions on your own. You will need to buy books that will help you with your studies.

Go to the Elsevier website and buy the online products you need. Help yourself out. Take that initiative. The secret to getting the HESI (Health Education Systems Incorporated) and NCLEX questions correct is to practice a lot of questions. You will need to combine studying the core content with developing your skills in answering questions. I advise that you get the adaptive quizzing resources for any Med-Surg book you are using in class. They will help you tremendously, especially in the area of 'multiple select' questions. Make sure that you are up to par in your studies. Never have a laissez-faire attitude towards your studies because if you lag behind in your studies you will most likely end up failing your exam. It can be very dangerous if you continue in this manner because you may never catch up. You can also surf the internet when studying. Use YouTube to check out study skills as well as lectures that you did not understand in class. There are good videos out there that will help you tremendously. You have to put a lot of hours into studying to make sure that you get the output you need, which is passing your exam in flying colors.

Chapter Eight

HONOR SCHEDULES BY BEING PUNCTUAL TO CLASS AND CLINICAL

Let me forewarn you that nursing school has zero tolerance for lateness and absenteeism, you need to check out your school policies in regards to those. The nursing program becomes your universe once you enroll in the school, everything you do rallies around it. Punctuality to class and clinical and submitting assignments on time are key priorities. The program requires you to be punctual in all that you do, ranging from your studies to your assignments and attendance to class whether it is in person or online due to the pandemic, and clinical. Let me forewarn you that you will have tons of assignments to complete and at the same time chapters of text books that you will need to finish reading in preparation for an exam. You must honor each schedule presented to you by being punctual.

You will constantly feel overwhelmed. The feeling of being overwhelmed will be very real to you, but know that it serves to test how well you are able to cope under pressure. As a nurse, you will be placed in charge of several patients. Your future employer would like to know that you will be punctual to work and will be able to take the pressure of dealing with patients and handling any emergency that comes your way. This is why nursing school is such a good training ground for developing the skills you will need as a professional nurse. If you are someone who is usually late, you need to change that attitude. If you do not, depending on the school policies you might be at risk for being expelled from the nursing program that you fought so hard to get into.

In the event you find out that you are running late to clinical for any reason or due to circumstances beyond your control, please have the courtesy of calling your instructor to inform him or her. The worst punishment you will suffer in such a situation is that you will be sent home for arriving late. If that occurs, please do not be that student who takes it out on the instructor. Remember that the instructor is also following rules and guidelines established for instructors. We all know that things happen in life that may cause you to be late. Even if you are sent home in such situations, your instructor will still give you make-up assignments to enable you complete your clinical hours. Please make sure you do them and submit them promptly. If you do not, you will be given a zero grade for that rotation which is not what you want (the policy may vary from school to school). This would portray that you are not a serious student. It would also, show that you are not prepared to take your responsibilities as a future nurse seriously. You must demonstrate that you are capable of being a nurse who is a good patient advocate and who will uphold the principles of non-maleficence and not allow any harm to befall the patient.

Chapter Nine

YOU SHALL NOT MISS CLINICAL UNLESS FOR VERY SERIOUS, GENUINE REASONS

Clinical, yeah! The following tips are very, very important. Do not underestimate what traffic or the weather will be like on the day of clinical. Be proactive. Always look up weather and traffic reports ahead of time. Make sure your car is serviced before the semester starts. You do not want to run into any problems on the day of clinical. There is no excuse that will warrant your absence from clinical except in the occurrence of death or in the occurrence of a critical situation. Even with that you can only have one absence on your record, if you are absent a second time you will be kicked out of the program. You might need to check your school policies on this, because it might vary from school to school. According to school policies and procedures, if you come in late to clinical you might be turned back and will have to make up for the hours you missed by doing lots of assignments. It is better for you not to miss or show up late to clinical at all. The semester is long and you can never tell what will happen in the future. You never know what emergency could arise. Therefore, I would encourage you not to take the risk of missing clinical or showing up late. Many people tried to get into the nursing program but could not. However, you have been given that opportunity. Make adequate use of the opportunity and come out with flying colors.

During clinical rotations you will receive hands-on experience in a hospital setting. This knowledge is invaluable. You will learn to relate to your patients, practice making-full head-to-toe assessment of patients, and administer medications under the supervision of your instructor as defined by hospital policies and procedures. You will get to demonstrate the skills taught by taking care of your patients and making use of your clinical judgment. There is a wealth of information to be acquired during clinical rotations. I would advise every student to be religiously punctual to clinical. The nursing program has zero tolerance for absenteeism. The board of nursing requires students to meet a certain number of hours in the completion of their degree program. If you miss a clinical day, you will miss out on required clinical hours. You will have to make up for all those hours you missed by completing make-up assignments which you will still be obligated to finish on time in addition to all the work you already have lined up for you. You do not want to go through this because you already have a lot of reading to do. If it is inevitable for you to miss a clinical day, let your instructor know. However, I would advise that you try as much as possible to be present and on time.

Make sure you prepare all the materials you will need for your clinical day the night before. Make sure you do not forget your school badge on clinical day as you will be turned away if you do and will miss clinical for that day. This is very risky. I would like to make one very important point here. Be sure to carry all the materials you need with you into the hospital before the start of clinical on the day of clinical. Once clinical sessions begin, you will not be allowed to leave the hospital units to retrieve any materials from your car.

Chapter Ten

YOU SHALL NOT SUBMIT YOUR ASSIGNMENTS EVEN A SECOND LATE

When assignments are given, if possible try to finish them way ahead of time. It helps to be one step ahead at all times. I would finish my assignments before the due date and if possible submit them before time. If not, I would wait until the due date to submit them. Please, please, please **DO NOT SUBMIT YOUR ASSIGNMENTS LATE** (not even a second late)! You may end up getting a zero in that class. That is a failing grade. If you are unfortunate to have that happen to you, do not take it personally and think that the professor does not like you. Remember that you are required to follow strictly the instructions given you. Do not give the instructor the opportunity to implement rules that would be detrimental to your goals. The nursing profession requires you to be disciplined.

I cannot stress the importance of assignments enough. You must not only submit your assignments on time. It is imperative that you also do well on your assignments. I advise that you strive towards making a hundred percent on all your assignments. These are the scores you will use to raise your grade in the event you do not do well on your exams. From experience, I can tell you that you are better off not failing an exam. The make-up assignments you will be given to improve your grade will add more workload to your reading. Remember that you already have a heavy workload.

Map out a comprehensive strategy that will help you meet your goals in nursing school. Buy yourself a pocket calendar and write down the due dates for all assignments. Set an alarm on your phone a day before each assignment is due to remind you that you have an assignment due the next day. Also, it pays to be ahead on assignments. Do them ahead of time and you will be alright. In the event you have difficulty with any assignment, remember that you have access to your instructor and your academic advisor. You can always set up an appointment with them and they will help you in your area of difficulty. You can also approach colleagues who you have observed to be helpful.

Chapter Eleven

YOU SHALL TACKLE AND REVIEW
MANY SAMPLE QUESTIONS

It is imperative to review NCLEX-style questions. This is one important strategy you should adopt to ensure success. Nursing school questions are rarely direct. They are tricky. You will be given scenarios or hypothetical situations to consider. Questions will be framed on those scenarios and with each question multiple answers will be provided. Sometimes all the answers may be right, but one of them would be the most accurate. The secret to answering a question correctly lies in knowing which multiple-choice answer is the most accurate. That is where knowing your content completely comes into play.

I encourage you to get the adaptive quizzing resources on the textbooks you are using at school. To educate yourself on what the best resource tools are, I hope you inquire more about the study materials other people use than I did during my time in nursing school. I only found out about the adaptive quizzing resources after the second to last exam of my final year. I started asking questions because the number of multiple-select questions on the exams had increased and I had difficulty with them. It finally occurred to me to ask a colleague what resources she was using to prepare for exams. That was how I found out about adaptive quizzing. Apparently, with multiple choice questions you can easily choose the correct answer if you know the content. However, with multiple select you have to be very certain what the correct answer is or you will end up choosing the wrong answer, meaning you will end up selecting your answer from the set of wrong choices or less accurate options provided.

I advise that you acquire other **NCLEX** books by authors like Hogan and Silvresti. Any Saunders resource book is good study material. These books give insight on how to answer questions correctly and how to develop your critical thinking ability. There are also online reviews that you can buy from resource providers like Elsevier, Lippincott, Kaplan or UWorld. When preparing for the HESI exit exam, you can obtain good resource material from resource providers like "Your Best Grade" and "Exam Edge". When studying, make sure you read the rationales for which particular answers are assigned to given questions. Going over the rationales is vital to understanding why the answer assigned to a given question is correct (that is, why it was selected over the other options provided). Rationales help you think critically about the reasons why certain actions are taken.

For example, you may be given a question with the following scenario:

Mr. B has just undergone cataract surgery and is ready to be discharged. Which of the following instructions will the nurse provide in terms of priority teaching?

A. Cover your eyes while sleeping

B. Do not put eye drops in the affected eye

C. Avoid coughing

D. Have someone help you ambulate

The correct answer is: *C. Avoid coughing.* Why? The rationale behind avoiding coughing is to prevent intraocular pressure.

Most schools incorporate the **HESI** exit exam into the final exam of the last semester in your final year and others don't, so find out how your school operates with the **HESI** exit exam. In that case, you will need to be prepared for the **HESI** exam as well. There are several books that will educate you on what to expect on the exam. I encourage you to get the necessary resources to enable you prepare in the most efficient way. Use the study aids wisely and apply yourself diligently to ensure success. You will definitely feel exhausted and burnt out. It is part of the nursing school experience. Know however, that whatever has a beginning will also have an end. *Perseverance* is the key, so **PRACTICE, PRACTICE, PRACTICE!**

Chapter Twelve

REMEMBER TO ASK QUESTIONS WHEN YOU DON'T UNDERSTAND

Remember to ask questions when you do not understand. Do not underestimate the benefit of questions because when you ask questions you get information and information is power. Once you get the information you need it will empower you to achieve your goal. Do not be timid. Never ever feel shy to ask questions in class or outside of class, no matter how stupid you think a question is, as far as it relates to the content you are covering. Some classmates may make you feel like you are asking too many questions, or that you would not have those questions if you had read the content. Maybe they understood the content but you did not. Remember that each person is different. We take exams individually. If that content comes up in the exam, you are the one who will have to answer the question so do not feel self-conscious. Just ask the question you desire and the teacher will answer you. I remember one time I had asked a question in class on content I had read but did not understand. One of my classmates had the audacity to comment, "Olivia, you should have read about this before class." I turned to her and said, "I did read about it but I still have a question to ask the instructor." Then, I went ahead and continued with my question from the point at which I had stopped when she interrupted me, and my question was answered.

You have every right to ask questions when you do not understand the content. The instructor will answer you. Also, when studying with your friends do not hesitate to ask questions because it helps to hear someone else talk about a topic. That discussion will most likely stick in your memory and during the exam when you see a question related to that subject you will recollect the conversation. Knowledge is power. Strive to get answers to all the questions that you have on content that you do not understand. Use different resources on the internet like YouTube and the website 'allnurses.com'. Google any information you need. You will be surprised to find an answer to every query you have. What I would do while studying was to have my YouTube page open. For example, in order to gain understanding on the topic of 'glomerulonephritis', I went on YouTube and typed 'glomerulonephritis for nurses' into the search bar. This brought up many videos on the subject. I watched a few of them and gained better understanding of the content I was covering at the time. You can search out any topic on the internet to learn more about it. You will understand it better in the end. The ball is in your court; be smart and play the game in such a way that you will score all the goals you need to win.

Chapter Thirteen

YOU SHALL FIND POSITIVE WAYS TO TAKE GOOD CARE OF YOURSELF AND MAINTAIN GOOD HEALTH DURING THE COURSE OF THE PROGRAM

I implore you to find positive ways to take good care of yourself in order to maintain good health. I really mean it. You need to take very good care of yourself during this period. Eating healthy and exercising are key factors in maintaining good health. Please stay away from junk food. Eat lots of fruits and vegetables and drink lots of water to hydrate your system. Be forewarned that you will be highly stressed out which would make you immunosuppressed and vulnerable to infections. To prevent yourself from getting sick, you need to eat healthy and maintain standard health precautions by washing your hands thoroughly and frequently to avoid self-contamination. Remember that you cannot afford to be sick at this time. If you are infective you will not be allowed to attend class or clinical. This would force you to be absent and you can only afford to miss a clinical day twice per semester, you will be kicked out of the program after that. At least that was the case with the nursing school I attended.

Everyone knows nursing school is tedious. The stress of nursing school is inevitable. To relieve stress, you will need to find a relaxing technique that works for you. My decompression techniques for tension are meditation, swimming, dancing and getting a massage. You need to find what works best for you and implement it. When you are tense, you often experience stiffness of muscle. It is very uncomfortable to have stiff muscles; you will need to properly address this if you experience it. Take thirty minutes out of your busy schedule and go for a massage to get the knots and tightness out of your muscles, if you are one for massages. Another technique that helps is doing deep breathing exercises that will help you breathe better. Most importantly, always remember to smile. Smiling takes a lot of tension off your system. In addition to having good nutrition or maintaining a healthy diet, you may need to include supplemental vitamins to your routine as this helps to boost your immune system. When out in the sun, always remember to hydrate. Drink lots of water. You can also fill up on sports drinks which promote hydration and help balance the electrolytes in your system. Sometimes, you can treat yourself to a relaxing bubble bath to really soothe you. Use any method that works for you − whether it is yoga, dance, exercise, meditation, music or reading, to mention a few.

Chapter Fourteen

FINAL SEMESTER

The final semester will be contrary to what you expect. The fact that you have excelled in so many class exams and are finally a senior could make you think you have got a hang of things. But surprise, surprise! Final semester classes are the hardest classes to pass. You must definitely have your game gear on. Without a doubt, you should continuously review your studying strategy to make sure you are studying the right way. If your previous strategy is not working, change it. If you have friends and colleagues who are excelling more than you are, do not hesitate to ask them how they study. Try to incorporate their style into your own study style to see if you can benefit from it. Please note that this is a critical time and not a time to be self-conscious or proud. Have an open mind and do not come out as if you know it all, because you could miss out on so much strategic information that could help you excel.

I encourage team or group work – only when you have finished studying on your own, otherwise you would be wasting your time. You would also be wasting the group's time. If you attend a study group without first studying, you will feel lost during the session. The members of the group might also not like the fact that you are not contributing. I will reiterate that it is vital for the group to assign reading chapters to all the group members.

By your final semester, your critical thinking skills would be well developed and you would be able to efficiently apply your knowledge of the content you have assimilated to any given question. In addition to your class work, it is imperative that you practice a lot of questions on your own. If you can afford it, register for online HESI practice exams with practice test providers like "Saunders' HESI Online Review", "Your Best Grade" or "Exam Edge" which all focus on the **HESI** exit exam. For the **NCLEX**, there are similar avenues with **UWORLD**, Hurst Review, Kaplan and many more. If you do not have money for the full package, you could get the test bank for one month and review it. The key to the final semester is to **PRACTICE, PRACTICE, PRACTICE.** Time management is vital. If possible, do your assignments ahead of time and strive to remain afloat and not get overwhelmed. Personally, I became so overwhelmed that one day I completely forgot that I had to go to class. I woke up tired and I relaxed in bed, my brain did not communicate that I had to be in school. Usually if am not in school I should be at work, but I did not ask myself why I was in bed. This incident occurred because I believe my system had shutdown. Somehow, later on, my brain knew that I had to do my pre-simulation (**SIM**) assignment but there was no communication within me whatsoever that I had to be in the Simulation Lab that day. Thus, I went about my day busy studying and then proceeded to do my pre-**SIM** assignment. I was able to do that successfully. However, when I tried to log into the system again later that day to do the post-**SIM** assignment the system would not let me in. I emailed my instructor to let her know I was not able to get in. I even went to the extent of calling Elsevier whose platform our coursework runs on and was told I could not get in because my instructor had locked students out of the system. The instructor had blocked student access because she had cancelled the post-SIM assignment for that day. We were no longer required to do it. Obviously, I was not aware of this since I did not attend class that day. I had missed Simulation Lab earlier without knowing it. The stress I was under at the time had thrown me off balance. I did not realize that I had missed SIM until evening when my colleagues inquired why I was not in class. What happened to me was very risky because the regulations state that if you miss more than two classes you will be kicked out of the program.

I believe my system had shut down and there was nothing I could do about it. I missed class and ended up having to do a lot of make-up assignments. I caved under the pressure of nursing school and my normal rhythm of doing things was completely thrown off. This goes to show that we can break down. It is important to eat well, exercise and hydrate our system, and believe it or not, find a little time to relax. All this will contribute to a person's overall wellbeing and boost academic performance. You need a firm understanding of how best to thrive in nursing school.

One important resource that a good number of students fail to utilize is the help of professors. If you have any questions, do not hesitate to ask your instructor. Instructors are very good at helping students and they are extremely knowledgeable in their field. They will give you good hints or advice on how to study effectively and how to apply your critical thinking abilities.

There is no greater joy than the day you take your final exam and look at your grade and find out you have passed. The euphoria is unimaginable. You feel like a great weight has been lifted off your shoulders. You feel like you are dreaming and will eventually wake up and reach for your Medical-Surgical book and start reading all over again. But the good thing is that it is real; your hard work has paid off. The ultimate goal is to pass the final semester and graduate.

Below are the messages a couple of my nursing school colleagues posted the day they found out they had passed the final exam, am including these with their permission.

"Well, It's OFFICIAL! I am a NURSING SCHOOL

GRADUATE! I'm DONE! This last semester was a toughie but I managed to hang in there. It just goes to show that if you truly want something, you WON'T give up. Only a handful of people know the struggles I faced trying to get where I am now. I've been through hell and back but I managed to keep my chin up and persevere. God has rewarded me! I know its late notice but for anyone interested, my pinning ceremony is tomorrow. If you'd like to cheer me on as I get formally welcomed into the nursing profession, PM me for details! #GoodByeNursingSchool#IDidIt#GraduateNurse#Next Stop NCLEX#FutureRN#

Erin C.

"After all the blood, sweat, and tears (literally... lol), the endless hours of studying, test anxiety and rough days when I felt like giving up...I can officially say I graduated nursing school!! Just passed my HESI RN exit exam and words can't express how happy I am!! Now onto the Boards but until then...celebration time!! #GraduateNurse#SoonToBeRN#oncloudnine#

Sara J.

There were so many other similar messages from my colleagues stating that their joy was inexpressible. No amount of words can express the joy that you will feel the day you realize you have passed. If you are fortunate enough to share in this experience, this is what I have to say to you: Well, congratulations new graduate nurse!

Hello! The big part is over. You are no longer worried about failing a class and having to repeat that class, or even repeating a class, failing it again, and then getting kicked out of the program. Now you have a bigger fish to fry and that is your NCLEX exam. This exam is a "must pass" exam. It is your key to being a registered nurse, so it is imperative that you pass it. Some people take time off after graduation before taking this exam and some people delve into it right away. It is advisable to take it right away after graduation as all the information you stored in your brain in studying for your final exam will still be fresh in your mind. However, if you feel burnt out and are not yet ready to take the board exam, take your time.

I do believe that anything worth doing is worth doing well. There is no rush, so take the exam at your own pace – when you are truly ready to take it. Be informed that the

NCLEX is comprehensive (like the HESI). It covers all the material that you were taught in nursing school.

As of the time this book was written, there are a minimum of seventy-five questions and a maximum of two hundred and sixty-five questions in an exam bank for the NCLEX exam. My advice for you is to take your time to review each question carefully before answering and clicking on the next button. Remember to understand each question and choose the correct answer before moving on to the next question. You have a timeframe of six hours for the exam. Your ultimate goal is not to finish the entire exam but to get the needed number of questions right to enable the grading system deem you knowledgeable enough to become a registered nurse.

You can do it. Yes, you can! I wish you all the best of luck in the Nursing Program and NCLEX!

Chapter Fifteen

NURSE RESIDENCY PROGRAM

I am incorporating this chapter because I deem it vital for the new graduate nurse to understand how imperative it is to get into the hospital residency program. This program is designed to train new nursing school graduates with hands-on or practical experience for a number of months. They are released onto the hospital floor under the supervision of a preceptor who oversees what they do. After your residency program, you will be released from this arrangement and will be on your own. However, most hospitals will make you sign a contract to stay with them for a specific timeframe before seeking employment elsewhere. It is an amazing opportunity which most hospitals have incorporated.

New graduates with a Bachelor of Science in Nursing (BSN) Degree can apply to any hospital for the residency program, but graduates with an Associate's Degree in Nursing (AND) will have to search for hospitals that are willing to employ them. I would advise you to seek admission into the RN-to-BSN Degree Completion Program in the final semester of your studies if you are in the RN program. It would give you an edge on your resume as hospitals you apply to would be more willing to hire you with an Associate's Degree knowing that you are in the process of getting your BSN. This is a good strategy since most hospitals are becoming magnet hospitals and are only allowed to employ nurses with the minimum qualification of a BSN.

My greatest challenge in nursing school occurred in my final semester when I ended up being completely burnt out. I had worked the whole time I was attending school and was able to manage my work and school schedule fairly well up until the last semester. In the last semester, my body began to shut down and I barely could study or understand what I was studying. I had to drag myself along and even happened to miss a clinical day for no reason. My system was not functioning at optimal level and I completely forgot I had to go to clinical. I made my worst grade in nursing school in my final semester. At a point, I thought I was going to fail but I managed to keep dragging myself along. I do believe that is the reason why most schools require students to do only 20 hours of work or less, check your school policy. I had to work because I had no helper or family around to depend on. Due to the way I felt at the time, I could only focus on passing my classes. I was not even ready to start applying to hospitals for my residency. That felt like extra work which I could not deal with at the time. After graduating, I did not take the **NCLEX**, the board exam, right away. I took some time off to recuperate and took the exam three months later. By the time I was physically ready to get into the residency program, the deadlines for most hospitals had passed. I have also found out that it is extremely difficult to get a nursing job when you are a new graduate as all the hospitals are looking for experienced nurses. I am incorporating an account of my experience to keep you informed. If I or any of my other classmates who did not apply for residency on time had known that there were specific times and application deadlines for the residency program, we would definitely have applied earlier. We did not apply because we did not know; we were informed by our instructors but were not aware of the deadlines for the applications.

In your last semester, I advise that you prepare your resume and start applying to residency programs in the hospitals of your choice. Do not wait until after you graduate. That way, once you are out of school you can immediately get into the program you desire. Hear it from one who has already experienced it: it is frustrating to be a registered nurse and not have a job. Please do not make the same mistake I made.

The good thing with applying to the residency program on time is that a hospital will hire you even before you take your **NCLEX**, based on the promise that you will take and pass your board exam as soon as possible. Just be aware of this possibility and always check when residency applications are open and what their deadlines might be.

Chapter Sixteen

FINANCIAL AID

There are financial obligations involved with pursuing the nursing program. You will need funds to cover school fees, lots of books, miscellaneous expenses, and medical attire like scrubs and appropriate shoes for clinical. During nursing school orientation, representatives from different departments in the school will inform you about the many available opportunities that you can benefit from. I advise that you pay close attention to the information provided in order to benefit fully from the resources available. Advisors from the Financial Aid Department will be present as well.

The amount of financial assistance you receive depends on your income and how many people are present in your household.

You may qualify for financial aid in the way of scholarships, grants, or subsidized and unsubsidized loans. In addition, investigate and consult resource centers within your town or city for other funding sources. For example, in Houston, Texas, the resource center Workforce Solutions is available to assist you with the information you need. Find out from your school who to speak to regarding Financial Aid. Book an appointment with a Financial Aid Advisor to discuss the options available to you. You may be required to provide pay stubs over a six-month period to verify your eligibility. There is no harm in trying. I advise that you avoid loans as much as you can and let them be your last resort. There are several scholarships that you can apply for. The financial assistance you receive will go a long way in offsetting some costs.

Chapter Seventeen

TESTIMONIES

I was very excited to get into nursing school, because I knew this is a rewarding career which is full of opportunities. I couldn't wait to see myself walking at graduation. However, nothing prepared me for the stress that I went through. The school program was very difficult, because there were simply too many materials you have to cover and then you have to prepare for exams within a short period of time. I made a decision that I will do all in my power to make it. So, I had to make study plan and studied little daily. I did not allow myself to waste any day without studying. I was very determined especially my last semester, because I had been fighting for this far. I basically calculated my grade averages every day to make sure I was on the right track. It definitely feels good to pass NCLEX, especially if you pass it on the first time. It was a huge relief because it was the ultimate goal you went to school for. Now you have the right to find a nursing job, so go for it! Make your resume look good and fill out as many job applications as you can. Also, if you have an ADN degree, try to get your BSN ASAP.

Will F, ADN, RN

Before choosing to pursue nursing as my second degree I had just finished with my first bachelors in psychology in pursuit of my masters. I have been working at a psychiatric hospital before coming to the realization that nursing was my calling. Once I found out that I had been accepted into nursing school I was so ecstatic. So much hard work placed in, and to finally get in was such a relief.

Nursing school was not that intense for me like many would think it is. Yes, it was tough and yes, it was demanding. But I believe because I had a foundation from my first degree that the shock wasn't as bad. Clinical was an adjustment and check off on skills were intense as well. But I wouldn't trade my time in nursing school for anything. The experience is like no other and it truly makes you realize the hard work we as nurses have to put in just to graduate.

When it came time to taking the NCLEX I was a total mess. I usually can keep a calm and cool demeanor when it came to taking an exam or anything with pressure generally. Studying for the NCLEX was extremely stressful. I had no direction in which to go and was basically studying blindly. The day of the exam I believe I took almost all of the allotted time because I wanted to make sure. My test shut off at 75 questions and I felt like I totally failed the exam. I was told by others that if you walk out with that feeling chances are you passed. I found out 2 days later (paid to find out earlier) that I was now a Registered Nurse with the State of Texas! It was the first step in my career.

-Carlos Contreras, BSN, RN

There is a phrase in Spanish that goes "Uno impone y

Dios dispone." It means that you can plan as much as you want, but sometimes life can take a turn you can never anticipate. While preparing for nursing school, I would spend countless hours imagining any possible scenario that could sabotage nursing school and find ways to solve them. I found myself comfortable, thinking that I had planned everything, and now all I had to worry about was passing the exams. Unfortunately, life had other plans for me.

I never considered being perfectly healthy one day, and the next day get diagnosed with stage 4 cancer. To say that my world got turned upside down is an understatement. Besides the dozens of questions I had about my prognosis, I needed to figure out what would happen to nursing school. I begged to be able to finish the semester, only to be told the cancer was so aggressive, I would not be alive by graduation. I needed to pause my plans, go through treatment, and return to school when I recovered.

I cried long and hard over pausing my studies because I wanted to stick to my plan. I felt defeated. All these feelings went away when I reached out to my professors and classmates. A massive wave of support surrounded me throughout my treatment and recovery. I never expected my professors and fellow nursing students would carry me through the way they did.

Everyone that is in the nursing field has one thing in common, and that is that we are nurturers. We have compassion. We have empathy. So, thinking back as to how they embraced me while I was in need, I wouldn't't have expected any less from them. While you are in nursing school, and really throughout all of your career, realize that you are there to support each other, to help each other grow. It is not a competition. Help others as you go through the program, but also let others help you.

You can plan and anticipate as much as you can imagine, but there may come to a point when you need others to help you achieve your goals or even keep your head above the water. You will be surprised how much further you can go when you all work together.

-Yashira Contreras, BSN, RN

The End